RESISTANCE DUMBBELL EXERCISES FOR SENIORS

Ultimate Workout Guide to Improve Flexibility, Muscle Strength, Balance, and Coordination

Emmanuel Klaver

COPYRIGHT 2023

ALL RIGHTS RESERVED

EMMANUEL KLAVER

Table of Contents

Introduction 8
    The Challenge of Aging 9
    Power of Exercise 10
    A Gentle Approach to Strength Training using Resistance Bands 11
    Building Strength with Precision using Dumbbells 11
    Safety First 12
    A Pathway to Active Aging 12

Need for Resistance Band and Dumbbell Exercises 14
    Muscle Strength and Mass Preservation: 14
    Improved Bone Density: 15
    Enhanced Joint Health: 15
    Maintaining Balance to Prevent Falls: 16
    Cardiovascular Health: 17
    Psychological Health: 17
    Social Interaction: 18
    Independence and Lifestyle Quality: 18

Factors to Consider 20
    1. Resistance Level: 20

2. Durability and Material: 20
3. Size and Length: 21
4. Grips and Handles: 21
5. Options for Anchoring: 22
6. Color Coding: 22
7. Storage and Mobility: 22
8. Allergies and Security: 23
9. Review and Reputation of the Brand: 23
10. Policy on Returns and Warranties: 23
11. Value and Cost: 24
12. Particular Use: 24

Nutrients Required 25
1. Carbohydrates: 25
2. Proteins: 25
3. Lipids (Fats): 25
4. Vitamins: 26
5. Minerals: 26
6. Water: 26
7. Fiber: 27
8. Antioxidants: 27
9. Essential Fatty Acids: 27
10. Amino Acids: 27

Resistance Band Exercises 29
Resistance Band Bicep Curls: 29

Resistance Band Seated Rows: 30
Resistance Bands Leg Extensions: 30
Resistance Bands Lateral Leg Raises: 31
Resistance Band Shoulder Press: 32
Resistance Bands Clamshells: 33
Resistance Band Tricep Extensions: 33
Resistance Band Torso Twists: 34
Resistance Band Seated Leg Curls: 35
Resistance Bands Chest Press: 35
Resistance Band Seated Leg Press: 36
Resistance Band Chest Flyes: 37
Resistance Band Hip Abduction: 38
Resistance Band Scapular Retraction: 38
Resistance Band Ankle Plantarflexion and Dorsiflexion: 39

Dumbbell Exercises 41
Dumbbells Bicep Curls: 41
Dumbbells Bent-Over Rows: 42
Dumbbells Leg Raises: 42
Dumbbells Lateral Raises: 43
Dumbbells Tricep Extensions: 44
Dumbbell Standing March: 44
Dumbbell Seated Leg Press: 45
Dumbbell Torso Twists: 46

Dumbbell Heel Raises: 46

Dumbbell Chest Press: 47

Dumbbell Step-Ups: 47

Dumbbell Pallof Press: 48

Dumbbell Wrist Flexion and Extension: 49

Dumbbell Wall Angels: 50

Dumbbell Farmer's Walk: 50

Effectiveness in Preventing Fall and Injuries 52

Conclusion 56

Introduction

Maintaining physical health and fitness becomes more crucial as we get older because aging is an unavoidable aspect of life. Like people of all ages, seniors can gain a lot from regular exercise to enhance their general wellbeing. Traditional exercise regimens, however, might not always be appropriate for seniors due to a variety of variables, such as joint problems, restricted mobility, or worries about damage.

This is where senior dumbbell and resistance band workouts come into play, providing a secure and reliable way to maintain your strength, health, and activity level.

The importance of senior fitness has just come to light, and with this understanding has come a change in training paradigms. Today, active aging is not only encouraged but also celebrated, and the days when elderly were restricted to rocking chairs are long gone.

This change is supported by an in-depth knowledge of the numerous physical and psychological advantages exercise has for the senior population.

Dumbbells and resistance bands have become two adaptable and affordable tools for seniors looking to start a structured workout program. These tools enable older persons to carry out a variety of exercises that are tailored to their unique requirements and limits without the need for sophisticated gym equipment or a strenuous exercise regimen.

With an emphasis on their benefits, safety precautions, and the many ways they can improve older people's life, this introduction attempts to provide a thorough review of resistance band and dumbbell workouts specifically designed for seniors.

The Challenge of Aging

Our bodies naturally change as we age, and these changes can have a significant impact on our physical capabilities. Bone density may decline, joints may stiffen, and balance may become affected as muscle mass tends to decline. Age-related illnesses including osteoporosis, arthritis, and heart disease can also make leading an active lifestyle more challenging.

It's important to keep in mind, nevertheless, that seniors are not helpless when it comes to fitness despite these difficulties. In actuality, maintaining an active lifestyle becomes even more crucial to ward off these age-related changes and preserve a high quality of life.

Power of Exercise

Many of the problems brought on by aging can be successfully treated with exercise. It has the ability to increase bone density, muscle strength, cardiovascular health, and general mental health. Regular exercise can also improve flexibility, balance, and coordination, which lower the risk of fractures and falls concerns that are common among seniors.

In addition to its physical advantages, exercise can reduce stress, anxiety, and depressive symptoms, making life happier and more rewarding.

A Gentle Approach to Strength Training using Resistance Bands

Seniors can exercise their muscles safely and effectively by using resistance bands instead of the dangerous devices and heavy weights. While reducing the stress on joints and tendons, these elastic bands offer resistance through a range of motion, encouraging muscular development and endurance.

We'll look at how resistance bands can be used in senior fitness routines, including detailed instructions and highlighting exercises designed to increase stability, strength, and flexibility.

Building Strength with Precision using Dumbbells

Dumbbells, which are sometimes underrated in terms of their value for seniors, provide a flexible way to strengthen particular muscle groups and enhance general fitness. Dumbbells can assist seniors target muscles, improve balance, and stop muscle loss when used with the right form and resistance levels. In this lesson, we'll explore a variety of dumbbell exercises that were created especially for older citizens, with a focus on security and progressive progression.

Safety First

It is crucial to address safety issues before introducing elders to resistance band and dumbbell activities. Before beginning any new exercise program, seniors should speak with their doctors, especially if they have underlying medical concerns. Exercise can be done safely if the right warm-up and cool-down routines are followed, proper form is maintained, and the right resistance levels are used. Throughout this tutorial, we will offer advice on these vital safety precautions.

A Pathway to Active Aging

This thorough manual attempts to arm seniors with the information and resources they need to start along the path of active aging. This resource will serve as your guide whether you're an elderly person hoping to keep your independence, a caregiver looking for ways to improve the wellbeing of your loved ones, or a fitness fanatic ready to spread the word about the advantages of exercise to senior citizens.

We shall go further into the area of resistance band and dumbbell workouts for seniors in the chapters that follow. We'll cover a wide selection of fitness activities suitable for all physical ability levels. Together, we can realize the full potential of these straightforward yet transforming technologies, enabling seniors to benefit from a fit and active lifestyle well into their golden years and reap its numerous benefits.

Need for Resistance Band and Dumbbell Exercises

Numerous physical, psychological, and behavioral issues that have an immediate influence on the aging population highlight the importance of resistance band and dumbbell exercises for seniors. These activities completely meet these needs, making them an essential part of senior fitness programs. Let's explore the specific requirements for seniors' resistance band and dumbbell exercises:

Muscle Strength and Mass Preservation:

Need: Sarcopenia, a condition where muscular mass and strength naturally deteriorate as we age, is a problem. When muscle mass is lost, it can lead to decreased mobility, balance problems, and difficulties carrying out daily chores. To remain independent and active as they age, seniors must maintain their muscle mass and strength.

Solution: Strengthening muscles with resistance band and dumbbell exercises is controlled and progressive. These workouts encourage muscular growth, aiding seniors in fending off sarcopenia's effects. Seniors can regain and maintain the strength required for daily tasks like moving groceries, getting out of chairs, or climbing stairs by focusing on specific muscle groups.

Improved Bone Density:

Need: Seniors are particularly concerned about osteoporosis, a disorder marked by brittle bones. Increased bone fracture and injury risk might lead to decreased mobility and independence.

Solution: Using dumbbells to do weight-bearing workouts can help increase bone density and lower the risk of fractures. These workouts strengthen the skeletal system and promote bone remodeling, improving defense against problems associated with osteoporosis.

Enhanced Joint Health:

Need: Joint stiffness and pain that comes with aging can limit movement and promote a sedentary lifestyle.

Exercises that maintain joint health without aggravating joint issues are necessary for seniors.

Solution: While still offering a strenuous workout, resistance band workouts are easy on the joints. Seniors can use them to perform low-impact strength training, which helps to maintain joint flexibility and stability without placing undue stress on joints like the knees or hips. Dumbbell exercises can be modified to meet the specific needs of each joint, preserving range of motion and reducing joint pain.

Maintaining Balance to Prevent Falls:

Need: Seniors should be especially cautious about falls because they frequently cause serious injuries. For the purpose of avoiding falls and sustaining independence, maintaining balance and stability is essential.

Solution: Seniors can enhance their balance and coordination by performing exercises with a resistance band and dumbbells. The core muscles, which are crucial for maintaining stability while walking or standing, are the focus of these workouts. Seniors who have improved balance are less likely to fall and can confidently move about their surroundings.

Cardiovascular Health:

Need: The major cause of death among seniors is cardiovascular disease. To live a long and healthy life, maintaining heart health is essential.

Solution: Certain dumbbell and resistance band exercises can be modified to offer cardiovascular advantages. Exercises like resistance band aerobics and circuit training with dumbbells, for instance, can increase heart rate and thus cardiovascular fitness. By improving heart and circulation health, these workouts lower the risk of developing heart-related problems.

Psychological Health:

Need: For elders, mental health is just as crucial as physical health. Age-related increases in depression, anxiety, and stress can lower one's overall quality of life.

Solution: Regular exercise, especially dumbbell and resistance band exercises, has been shown to improve mood, lower stress levels, and lessen the effects of depression and anxiety. Exercise increases endorphin production, which improves cognitive performance and fosters a positive view on life.

Social Interaction:

Need: Seniors frequently experience social isolation, which can be harmful to their mental and emotional well-being.

Solution: Attending group fitness classes or working out with a friend can promote friendships and reduce loneliness. Exercises using resistance bands and dumbbells can be easily introduced into group sessions to encourage senior citizens' social interaction and sense of community.

Independence and Lifestyle Quality:

Need: Seniors who want to keep their independence and great quality of life in their later years would benefit most from resistance band and dumbbell exercises.

Solution: These exercises give seniors the freedom to live their lives on their terms by addressing the physical and psychological effects of aging. They make it possible for seniors to continue participating in social activities, carry out everyday tasks with ease, and feel in charge of their health and well-being.

Seniors who want to keep an active and independent lifestyle in their later years should engage in resistance band and dumbbell workouts. These exercises are not only optional parts of a fitness routine.

These exercises promote physical health, mental well-being, and social involvement while offering a comprehensive answer to the particular problems that elders encounter.

Adopting these exercises can result in a senior population that is happier, healthier, and more active.

Factors to Consider

It's crucial to take into account a number of aspects when selecting a resistance band to make sure you receive the one that best meets your fitness requirements and tastes. When choosing a resistance band, keep the following things in mind:

1. Resistance Level:

Resistance bands come in a variety of resistance levels, which are typically characterized by color or level of resistance (for example, light, medium, or heavy).

Pick a resistance band that is appropriate for the exercises you intend to do and your current level of fitness. It is preferable to begin with a lesser resistance band and increase the tension as necessary.

2. Durability and Material:

Latex, rubber, and cloth are a few of the materials commonly used to make resistance bands.

While rubber bands are popular, if you have a latex allergy you should think about alternatives.

Seek out bands with sturdy construction to make sure they won't shatter or break while being worn. Verify if the handles and seams are reinforced.

3. Size and Length:

There are many different sizes and lengths of resistance bands.

Longer bands can offer greater flexibility during exercises and a larger range of motion.

When selecting the length and size of your resistance band, take into account the activities you intend to undertake as well as the size of your body.

4. Grips and Handles:

While some resistance bands are just looped bands, others have handles or grips.

Handles can make it easier and more secure to hold an object during exercises that require pulling or pushing actions.

Ensure that the handles are soft and satisfying to hold.

5. Options for Anchoring:

Determine whether the resistance band has the proper attachments or accessories if you intend to use it for exercises that call for anchoring, such as door anchor exercises.

6. Color Coding:

To signify different resistance levels, many companies color-code their resistance bands.

Get acquainted with the brand's color coding system to make it simpler to determine the resistance level.

7. Storage and Mobility:

Take into account the resistance band's mobility. Choose a band that is small and convenient to store if you intend to use it both at home and elsewhere, such as the gym or when traveling.

8. Allergies and Security:

To prevent any negative reactions, select resistance bands without latex if you have a latex allergy.

Before each usage, check the band for flaws, cuts, or tears to make sure it's safe to wear.

9. Review and Reputation of the Brand:

To evaluate the strength and quality of the resistance band you're contemplating, do some brand research and read customer reviews.

A reliable product will be more likely to be offered by a reputable brand with favorable ratings.

10. Policy on Returns and Warranties:

Verify whether a warranty or satisfaction guarantee is offered with the resistance band.

Recognize the return policy in the event that the band falls short of your expectations or has manufacturing defects.

11. Value and Cost:

To make sure you're getting a decent deal for your money, compare costs across several brands and models.

Remember that purchasing a high-quality resistance band can be an affordable approach to keep up your fitness.

12. Particular Use:

Take into account the kinds of exercises you want to use the resistance band for. Consider a band that is waterproof or water-resistant if you intend to work out in the water, for instance.

Carefully taking into account these elements, you may choose a resistance band that is in line with your fitness objectives, preferences, and any unique needs you may have, ensuring a secure and efficient workout.

Nutrients Required

Your body requires nutrients in order to function properly and retain good health. They are separated into various types, each of which serves a particular purpose within the body. The following are the necessary nutrients and their roles:

1. Carbohydrates:

Function: The body uses carbohydrates as its main energy source. Your muscles and brain are fed by them.

2. Proteins:

Function: Proteins are necessary for the development, maintenance, and repair of tissues. They contribute to the manufacture of hormones, immunological response, and enzymes.

3. Lipids (Fats):

Function: Dietary lipids assist the body absorbs the fat-soluble vitamins A, D, E, and K, encourages cell growth, and provides energy. They contribute to the synthesis of hormones as well.

4. Vitamins:

Function: Vitamins are organic substances that are essential for a number of body processes. In addition to numerous other processes, they promote the immune system, metabolism, eyesight, and skin health. Vitamins can be classified as either water-soluble (B-complex vitamins or vitamin C) or fat-soluble (A, D, E, and K).

5. Minerals:

Function: Minerals, which are inorganic nutrients, are crucial for preserving health. They support iron transport, fluid balance (sodium, potassium), the health of the teeth and bones (calcium, phosphorus), and more.

6. Water:

Function: Water is necessary for almost all body processes. In addition to acting as a solvent and controlling body temperature, it also carries nutrition, eliminates waste, and cushions organs.

7. Fiber:

Function: Dietary fiber is a kind of carbohydrate that the body does not digest. It promotes heart health by decreasing cholesterol levels and aids in digestion, avoids constipation, and promotes digestion.

8. Antioxidants:

Function: Antioxidants, including the vitamins C and E, selenium, and a number of phytochemicals, aid in preventing free radical damage to cells. They contribute to improving general health and lowering the risk of chronic diseases.

9. Essential Fatty Acids:

Function: Omega-3 and omega-6 fatty acids are crucial for keeping healthy skin, hair, and the brain, as well as for lowering inflammation.

10. Amino Acids:

Function: Amino acids are the fundamental components of proteins. The body cannot synthesize several necessary amino acids, so we must consume them through diet. They are essential for the production of proteins and general health.

Depending on variables including age, gender, activity level, and individual health concerns, different nutrients may be needed at different times.

Supplements may be necessary in some situations for people to satisfy their nutritional demands, but it's important to speak with a healthcare provider before beginning any supplementation routine because an excessive amount of particular nutrients might have negative effects.

Resistance Band Exercises

Seniors might benefit greatly from using resistance bands in their training routines. They offer a secure and efficient technique to enhance fitness levels all around, including strength and flexibility. Here are 15 detailed resistance band workouts made especially for seniors:

Resistance Band Bicep Curls:

Muscles Targeted: Biceps brachii (Front of upper arm muscle)

Instructions:

1. Stand with your feet shoulder-width apart on the resistance band.

2. Hold the band with your arms fully extended and palms facing forward.

3. Slowly bend your arms, curving the band toward your chest while keeping your elbows close to your sides.

4. At the top of the curl, pause, and then gradually return the band to its starting position.

5. 2-3 sets of 10-15 reps should be done.

Resistance Band Seated Rows:

Muscles Targeted: Shoulders and upper back.

Instructions:

1. Legs extended, the band firmly fixed in front of you as you sit down on a chair.

2. Maintain a straight back while holding the band with both hands, palms facing one another.

3. Your shoulder blades should be squeezed together as you pull the band toward your torso.

4. Return to the starting posture after gradually releasing the tension.

5. 2-3 sets of 10-15 reps should be done.

Resistance Bands Leg Extensions:

Muscles Targeted: Quadriceps (front of thigh) muscles.

Instructions:

1. The band should be fastened behind you and around your ankles when you sit in a chair.

2. Flex the foot of the forward-extending leg.

3. Your knee should be straightened as you push against the band's resistance.

4. Bring your foot back to the starting position gradually.

5. Do 2-3 sets of 10-15 repetitions for each leg.

Resistance Bands Lateral Leg Raises:

Muscles Targeted: Hip and outer thigh abductors.

Instructions:

1. One end of the band should be fastened to a sturdy item, such as a table or chair leg.

2. Loop the other end around your ankle.

3. Hold onto a support for balance as you stand sideways to the anchor point.

4. In spite of the band's resistance, extend your leg while maintaining its straightness.

5. Returning to the beginning position, lower your leg.

6. Do 2-3 sets of 10-15 repetitions for each leg.

Resistance Band Shoulder Press:

Muscles Targeted: Deltoids (shoulder muscles).

Instructions:

1. Place the band firmly beneath your feet when you sit down on a chair.

2. Hold the band handles with your palms facing forward at shoulder height.

3. Up till your arms are fully extended, push the handles upward.

4. Return your arms to shoulder height gradually.

5. 2-3 sets of 10-15 reps should be done.

Resistance Bands Clamshells:

Muscles Targeted: Gluteus medius (outer hip).

Instructions:

1. Legs should be 90 degrees bent while you lay on your side.

2. The resistance band should be placed directly above your knees.

3. Keep your feet together while raising your top knee up against the band's resistance.

4. Returning to the starting posture, lower your knee down.

5. Do 2-3 sets of 10-15 repetitions on each side.

Resistance Band Tricep Extensions:

Muscles Targeted: Triceps brachii (behind of upper arm).

Instructions:

1. With one foot, stand on the resistance band.

2. With one hand raised overhead and an elbow bent, hold the band.

3. Straighten your elbow and fully extend your arm.

4. In order to get back to the starting position, slowly bend your elbow.

5. Do 2-3 sets of 10-15 repetitions on each arm.

Resistance Band Torso Twists:

Muscles Targeted: Obliques (side abdominal muscles).

Instructions:

1. The band should be secured behind you as you sit in a chair.

2. With both hands, hold the band handles close to your chest.

3. Turn your body to one side while maintaining a constant hip position.

4. After coming back to the center, turn to the opposite side.

5. 2-3 sets of 10-15 reps should be done on each side.

Resistance Band Seated Leg Curls:

Muscles Targeted: Hamstrings (back of thigh) muscles.

Instructions:

1. Place the band firmly beneath your feet when you sit down on a chair.

2. Your ankles should be wrapped with the band.

3. Flex your knee and, despite the band's resistance, push your heel up toward your glutes.

4. Return your leg to its initial position slowly.

5. Do 2-3 sets of 10-15 repetitions for each leg.

Resistance Bands Chest Press:

Muscles Targeted: Pectoralis major (chest muscles).

Instructions:

1. The band should be secured behind you as you sit in a chair.

2. Hold the band handles with your palms facing forward at chest height.

3. While extending your arms out in front of you, push the handles forward.

4. Return to the starting position gradually.

5. 2-3 sets of 10-15 reps should be done.

Resistance Band Seated Leg Press:

Muscles Targeted: Quadriceps (front of thigh), hamstrings (back of thigh), and glutes.

Instructions:

1. The resistance band should be wrapped around your feet as you sit in a chair with your back straight.

2. With your hands, hold the band's ends.

3. When your knees are fully extended, press your legs outward against the band's resistance.

4. Return to the starting posture after gradually releasing the strain.

5. 2-3 sets of 10-15 reps should be done.

Resistance Band Chest Flyes:

Muscles Targeted: Pectoralis major (chest muscles) and anterior deltoids (front shoulder).

Instructions:

1. Wrap the resistance band over your upper back while sitting in a chair and keeping the ends in each hand.

2. Start by extending your arms to chest height in front of you.

3. Squeeze your chest muscles while spreading your arms widely and extending the band.

4. Return to the starting position gradually while maintaining band tension.

5. 2-3 sets of 10-15 reps should be done.

Resistance Band Hip Abduction:

Muscles Targeted: Hip abductors (outer hip).

Instructions:

1. Connect the resistance band's one end to a sturdy object, such as a table or chair leg.

2. Your ankles will be encircled by the other end.

3. Hold onto a support for balance as you stand sideways to the anchor point.

4. Lift your outside leg while maintaining its straightness in the face of the band's opposition.

5. Returning to the beginning position, lower your leg.

6. Do 2-3 sets of 10-15 repetitions for each leg.

Resistance Band Scapular Retraction:

Muscles Targeted: Upper back and shoulder blade muscles.

Instructions:

1. Hold the resistance band in front of you with both hands while sitting or standing erect.

2. Continue to hold your arms out at shoulder level.

3. Pull the band apart while squeezing your shoulder blades together.

4. Hold the squeeze for a little period of time, then let go of the pressure to go back to the beginning position.

5. Complete 2-3 sets of 10-15 repetitions.

Resistance Band Ankle Plantarflexion and Dorsiflexion:

Muscles Targeted: Plantarflexion of the calves and dorsiflexion of the anterior shin muscles.

Instructions:

1. Place the resistance band around your feet while sitting on a chair with your back straight.

2. Hold the band's ends in your palms.

3. Point your feet away from you while pressing your toes downward to perform plantarflexion.

4. To perform dorsiflexion, raise your toes upwards while flexing your ankles in your direction.

5. Carry out 2-3 sets of 10-15 repetitions for each exercise.

Seniors can use these resistance band workouts to target various muscle areas, increase strength, and improve their overall functional fitness.

Also, remember to keep perfect form at all times.

Start with a comfortable amount of resistance and increase it gradually as your strength and confidence grow. Always use good form, and before starting your exercise program if you feel any pain or discomfort, speak with a medical practitioner or fitness professional.

Dumbbell Exercises

For seniors looking to increase their strength, flexibility, and general fitness, dumbbell workouts offer a flexible and efficient method. 15 comprehensive dumbbell exercises for seniors are listed below:

Dumbbells Bicep Curls:

Muscles Targeted: Front of upper arm muscle, biceps brachii.

Instructions:

1. Holding a dumbbell in each hand with your arms fully extended and palms facing forward, stand with your feet hip-width apart.

2. Curl the dumbbells toward your shoulders while slowly bending your elbows.

3. After a brief pause at the peak of the curl, lower the weights to the starting position.

4. Complete 2-3 sets of 10-15 repetitions.

Dumbbells Bent-Over Rows:

Muscles Targeted: Shoulders and the upper back.

Instructions:

1. Holding a dumbbell in each hand with your arms out in front of you, stand with your feet hip-width apart.

2. Keep your back straight and your chest up while bending slightly at the hips and knees.

3. Pull the dumbbells toward your torso while tightening the muscles in your shoulder blades.

4. While slowly lowering the weights back down, keep your posture straight.

5. Complete 2-3 sets of 10-15 repetitions.

Dumbbells Leg Raises:

Muscles Targeted: Quadriceps (front of thigh) muscles.

Instructions:

1. While holding a dumbbell at either side, stand with your feet hip-width apart.

2. Extend your leg forward while flexing one knee and raising your thigh until it is parallel to the ground.

3. Return your leg to its initial position.

4. Complete 2-3 sets of 10-15 repetitions for each leg.

Dumbbells Lateral Raises:

Muscles Targeted: Deltoids (shoulder muscles).

Instructions:

1. While holding a dumbbell at either side, stand with your feet hip-width apart.

2. While maintaining a slight bend in your elbows, raise your arms laterally to shoulder level.

3. After a brief minute of holding at the peak of the lift, bring your arms back to your sides.

4. Complete 2-3 sets of 10-15 repetitions.

Dumbbells Tricep Extensions:

Muscles Targeted: Triceps brachii (behind of upper arm).

Instructions:

1. Hold a dumbbell above with both hands while standing with your feet hip-width apart.

2. Lift the dumbbell up while keeping your arms fully extended and your elbows near to your ears.

3. To get back to your starting posture, slowly bend your elbows.

4. Complete 2-3 sets of 10-15 repetitions.

Dumbbell Standing March:

Muscles Targeted: The core, your balance, and your coordination.

Instructions:

1. While holding a dumbbell at either side, stand with your feet hip-width apart.

2. While extending the left arm, raise your right leg as high as is comfortable.

3. Return your arm and leg to their initial positions.

4. Repeat with the right arm and left knee.

5. Complete 2-3 sets of 10-15 repetitions for each leg.

Dumbbell Seated Leg Press:

Muscles Targeted: Quadriceps (front of thigh).

Instructions:

1. Place a dumbbell at your sides while seated on a chair with your back straight.

2. Stand with your feet hip-width apart and push your legs outward against the dumbbells' resistance.

3. Return to the beginning posture while gradually releasing the strain.

4. Complete 2-3 sets of 10-15 repetitions.

Dumbbell Torso Twists:

Muscles Targeted: Obliques (side abdominal muscles).

Instructions:

1. Hold a dumbbell in both hands and hold it near to your chest while sitting on a chair with your feet flat on the floor.

2. While maintaining a stationary hip position, rotate your torso to one side.

3. Turn to the opposite side after coming back to the center.

4. Complete 2-3 sets of 10 to 15 repetitions on each side.

Dumbbell Heel Raises:

Muscles Targeted: Calves.

Instructions:

1. While holding a dumbbell at either side, stand with your feet hip-width apart.

2. While balancing on the balls of your feet, lift your heels as high as is comfortable.

3. Lower your heels to the floor.

4. Complete 2-3 sets of 10-15 repetitions.

Dumbbell Chest Press:

Muscles Targeted: Pectoralis major (chest muscles).

Instructions:

1. Place a dumbbell at chest level in each hand while sitting on a chair with your back straight.

2. While fully extending your arms in front of you, push the dumbbells forward.

3. Take it slowly back to where you were.

4. Complete 2-3 sets of 10-15 repetitions.

Dumbbell Step-Ups:

Muscles Targeted: Quadriceps (front of thigh), hamstrings (back of thigh), and glutes.

Instructions:

1. Hold a dumbbell in each hand at your sides while you stand in front of a sturdy chair or step.

2. Place one foot on the step or chair and lift your body by pressing through your heel.

3. While erect on the step, extend your hip and knee fully.

4. Retract your steps and extend the opposite leg.

5. Complete 2-3 sets of 10-15 repetitions for each leg.

Dumbbell Pallof Press:

Muscles Targeted: Stabilizers, the core, and the obliques (side abdominal muscles).

Instructions:

1. Fasten a resistance band to an anchor point that is reliable.

2. While standing sideways to the anchor, hold a dumbbell in both hands at chest height.

3. Fully extend your arms, pushing the dumbbell away from your chest and buckling against the band's pull.

4. As you bring the dumbbell back to your chest, keep your balance and composure

5. Complete 2-3 sets of 10-15 repetitions on each side.

Dumbbell Wrist Flexion and Extension:

Muscles Targeted: Forearm flexors and extensors.

Instructions:

1. Hold a dumbbell in each hand while seated on a chair with your forearms resting on your thighs and palms facing up.

2. Lift the dumbbells toward your body while flexing your wrists, and then stretch your wrists by lowering them near your knees.

3. To strengthen your wrists, perform 2-3 sets of 10-15 repetitions.

Dumbbell Wall Angels:

Muscles Targeted: Upper back and shoulder mobility and stability.

Instructions:

1. Hold a dumbbell in each hand while maintaining a 90-degree angle with your arms while standing with your back against a wall.

2. Slide your arms up and down the wall while keeping your wrists, elbows, and back in touch.

3. Maintain an engaged core and concentrate on good posture.

4. Complete 2-3 sets of 10-15 repetitions.

Dumbbell Farmer's Walk:

Muscles Targeted: Core stability, grip strength, and overall body strength.

Instructions:

1. Stand holding a dumbbell in each of your side-facing hands.

2. Carry the dumbbells and advance with short, controlled steps.

3. Maintain a tight core and a straight back.

4. Walk a certain distance or amount of time before going back to where you started.

5. Carry out 2-3 sets of farmer's walks, progressively extending the distance or duration.

These workouts provide seniors a well-rounded workout by working different muscle groups and enhancing their overall strength, balance, and functional fitness.

Always start with a weight that you can bear easily and progressively raise it as your strength improves.

Effectiveness in Preventing Fall and Injuries

Exercises with resistance bands and dumbbells can be quite beneficial in lowering senior citizens' risk of falls and injuries. The following are some ways that using these exercises in a regular fitness regimen might help to improve balance, strength, and fall prevention in general:

1. Increased Muscle Strength: Dumbbell and resistance band workouts target a variety of muscle groups, including those in charge of maintaining stability and balance.

Seniors who exercise their legs, hips, and core muscles have better control over their movements and are less likely to stumble or lose their balance.

2. Better Balance and Coordination: Many exercises with resistance bands and dumbbells call for careful, controlled movements, which can improve balance and coordination.

Performing balance-focused activities, such as leg lifts or bicep curls while standing on one leg, challenges stability and improves balance in seniors.

3. Enhanced Bone Density: Dumbbell lunges and squats can help enhance bone density, which lowers the chance of fractures in the event of a fall.

Stronger bones are less prone to break under impact.

4. Enhanced Joint Flexibility: Exercises with resistance bands, in particular, encourage joint flexibility and range of motion.

Seniors who have more mobile joints can react to sudden movements and keep their balance better.

5. Postural Benefits: Exercises with a resistance band and dumbbells promote better posture, which is essential for preserving stability.

Through optimal alignment of the body's center of gravity, improved posture lowers the risk of falls.

6. Functional Strength: By enhancing functional strength, these workouts will help you do daily tasks like walking, climbing stairs, and lifting things more effectively.

Seniors develop greater self-assurance in their physical prowess and are less likely to have mishaps while going about their everyday business.

7. Fall Recovery Skills: Strength and conditioning developed through resistance band and dumbbell workouts can help with getting up after stumbling or coming close to falling. Seniors with stronger muscles are better able to maintain their balance after a fall and have a lower risk of suffering catastrophic injuries.

8. Enhanced Confidence: Seniors who regularly engage in strength and balance activities may feel more confident in their physical capabilities.

A more active and engaged lifestyle can result from decreased fear of falling and increased confidence.

9. Lower Risk of Chronic illnesses: Regular exercise, such as resistance band and dumbbell exercises, can help manage chronic illnesses including osteoporosis, arthritis, and diabetes, which can increase the Risk of Falling.

10. Personalized Approach: Seniors who use resistance bands and dumbbells can modify the workouts to suit their own requirements and capabilities, making it a flexible and personalized method of preventing falls.

Conclusion

Seniors' life can be changed by resistance band and dumbbell workouts, which provide a way to enhance their strength, balance, and general well-being. These straightforward yet efficient instruments may hold the secret to a life marked by self-assurance, independence, and a lower chance of accidents and slips and falls.

Seniors can strengthen their muscles, improve their coordination, and increase their bone density by committing to regular exercise. These advantages not only reduce the chance of falls but also give them the ability to recover quickly in the event of a stumble. Seniors who enjoy an active lifestyle and have better posture and self-confidence can enjoy the independence of carrying out regular tasks with ease.

Seniors must understand that starting a path to greater health and fall prevention can never be too late. Resistance bands and dumbbells' adaptability enables exercises to be customized for specific needs and allows for pleasant advancement. To ensure safety and suitability for particular health issues, it is imperative to obtain advice from medical specialists or fitness experts.

Seniors' dumbbell and resistance band exercises are ultimately more than just physical routines; they are a way to live a life that is strong, resilient, and full of life. Seniors can unleash the potential for a healthier, more active and fulfilling life by embracing these tools and committing to a routine of regular exercise, guaranteeing that every day is a step towards a brighter and more secure future.

SELF REFLECTION QUESTIONS

1. What are the Difficulties or Challenges you are currently facing? And how do plan on getting it solved by using this book?

2. How do you feel towards the exercises explained in this book? And do you believe it will help you in solving your problem?

3. Do you see this book as being self-explanatory?

4. Do you notice any progress when exercising?

5. Being a senior, what is your best exercise in the resistance band?

6. Being a senior, what is your best exercise in the Dumbbell section?

7. How was the overall experience?

8. Did you exercise with your partner? How was his/her experience?

NOTES

NOTES

NOTES

NOTES

NOTES

Milton Keynes UK
Ingram Content Group UK Ltd.
UKHW022047121224
3628UKWH00057B/2592